HOME EXERCISES FOR GOOD POSTURE:

Good posture means good looks and good health

Best Exercises for good posture in the privacy of your own home. You do not have to go to the gym or buy expensive equipment to exercise for good posture!

BY   S. ELIA

DISCLAIMER:
This book is for information only. If you have any
health problems with your spine or any other
health issues please   consult your trusted doctor
before starting any vigorous exercises.

INTRODUCTION

Some people are blessed with a natural good posture and others have to exercise hard to get a good posture. Sometimes it is in the genes inherited from their ancestors and sometimes a good posture is due to good postural habits during their early days from infancy to adulthood. They were taught by their parents and mentors either at home or school how to sit properly, how to walk right , how to avoid bad sitting positions and how to avoid injury to their spines by bending and lifting the right way. Bad sitting positions can cause problems to the spine leading to scoliosis, kyphosis, lordosis and a bad posture.

The spine is the key for a good posture. A straight spine without any abnormal spinal curves is the key for a perfect posture. For anybody that wants to have a good posture it is necessary to take good care of their spine and do the right exercises to develop a strong , healthy and flexible spine. Anybody can have a good posture but they have to be willing to work for it. Unfortunately they did not invent a magic pill for a perfect posture and it is unlikely that they will ever invent one. A bad Posture is a structural problem and not a disease to cure it with pills. The only way to have a good posture is to work for it, period.

Many people are just wishing to have a good posture but they fail to do anything about it. If you are serious about improving your posture, you have to start doing the right exercises today, NOW, not tomorrow, not next week, not when you have the time. If you want to improve your posture you will find the time, at home at work, anywhere you are , you will be thinking and acting upon attaining a good posture.

What is a good posture anyway.

Posture is the position you hold your body upright while standing, sitting, walking and lying down. A good posture is when your body is straight with your shoulders back , your abdomen in and your chin up and you look straight from any angle.. Ballerinas usually have a good graceful posture due to their long arduous training. Like ballerinas and soldiers, Good posture involves training your body to stand, walk, sit and lie in comfortable positions where the least strain is placed on your joints, muscles and ligaments during movement or weight-bearing activities. Hard work and training with the right exercises has its rewards, a good posture , self-confidence , good looks that

naturally exudes an aura of assertiveness and sex
appeal.
So I think it is worth the effort to exercise for a
good posture.

Benefits of a Good Posture

The benefits of good posture are many and
self satisfying.
How you look and feel is directly related to your
posture, improves your image , your good looks,
your self-confidence and makes you more
attractive.
Having a good posture is more than looking good,
It helps you to develop strength, flexibility, and
balance in your body. With good posture you have
less muscle pain and more energy throughout the
day. Proper posture also reduces stress on your
muscles and ligaments,   and reduces the risk of
injury and disease.

**With good posture you Avoid health
complications and your muscles, joints,
ligaments, and all the organs of the body work
properly.**
 A bad posture results in several health
complications over time, such as scoliosis,

kyphosis, lordosis, increased risks of slipped and
degenerated spinal discs, arthritis, spinal injuries,
back aches,   chest pains, breathing problems, poor
blood circulation and other health problems..

How to Improve Your Posture

  If you want to have A good posture you have to
work for it and eliminate any bad habits that
promote bad posture. This includes bad postural
habits at home watching TV,, reading while lying
down,   slouching, and sleeping on your stomach .
Good posture aligns everything in your body,
Bones, muscles, ligaments and tendons are all able
to function optimally when you sit or stand up
straight. Your organs work properly with good
posture.
A person who slouches may find that bad posture
affects unfavorably their body   to function
properly and they may have problems with their
digestive system,   have difficulty breathing and
experience various aches and pains. These poor
habits create greater physical problems as the body
ages. that's why it is very important to learn how
to have better posture from an early stage.
It is advisable that the parents teach their kids by
example the importance of good posture from an

early age. Many kids consciously and subconsciously copy and mimic their parents habits. There is a saying " monkey see ,monkey monkey do" and that's true for the kids mimicking their parents habits both postural and verbal habits. Many kids develop spinal problems including scoliosis, kyphosis and lordosis from slouching and bad sitting habits at home and at school. Proper sitting posture is important for everyone, particularly those who work at a desk all day. Sedentary life can lead to bad posture and health problems, hence it is always advisable to have good chairs, sit right and to exercise daily to keep the body in good alignment and good posture.

THESE EXERCISES CAN HELP YOU HAVE A GOOD POSTURE.

There are many exercises that can help you achieve a good posture but you have to have the desire and willingness to work hard to achieve your goal, which is a good posture. Nobody can do theses exercises for you, you and only you must do these exercises daily for ever to achieve your desired goal.
Many of the exercises that can teach you how to fix your posture are easy to perform and don't require much in the way of equipment. This means that

you can discover how to improve your posture from the privacy of your home and without investing a lot of money. These posture exercises will help you reach a new level of health, a good posture and fitness. Like everything else Nothing comes easy and you have to work hard to achieve a good posture and reap the benefits that come along with a good posture, good looks, self-confidence, sex appeal and above all good health.

The best exercises for good posture are the ones used by the ballerinas training, the professional athletes, body builders and others that have good posture. However the purpose here is not to become ballerinas , body builders and professional athletes by spending a lot of time exercising but to do the right exercises to achieve a good posture in the minimum time possible without expensive equipment. You do not even have to go to the gym or hiring a personal trainer. You can do these exercises in the privacy of your home. All you need is your desire, will and determination to achieve your goal, a good posture. After doing the right exercises and getting a good posture, it will be natural for you to keep a good posture anytime anywhere in anything you do.

THE MAIN EXERCISES FOR GOOD POSTURE

 As I said before, before starting any exercises, you have to eliminate your bad habits that prevent you from having a good posture. The habits that prevent most of the people with bad posture from having a good posture are the following. Slouching when you sit on the table to eat, slouching when you read, slouching when you sit at school in class, slouching when you play video games, slouching when you watch television or a movie, slouching at work and finally slouching when you stand and walk.
The number one enemy of good posture is SLOUCHING,.

A bad posture will give you a lot of health

problems, scoliosis, kyphosis, lordosis, pains and aches and as you get older you will have arthritis in your spine and other joints. So avoid slouching and you will be on your way for good posture and good health .

In my book SCOLIOSIS: HOW TO PREVENT AND TREAT SCOLIOSIS WITH HOME EXERCISES, available at amazon.com I explain in detail how to prevent spinal problems and get a good , strong and healthy spine which is prerequisite to have a good posture.

The spine is the key for a good posture and good health.

 Eliminate your bad habits of slouching and replace them with good postural habits and you are halfway through to a good posture. when you are sitting on a chair no matter where you are at school, home or work make it a habit to sit straight, never slouch even if you are bored. If you are tired or bored get up and walk.

When walking make it a habit to walk tall, with your body straight and never in a slouch position. Feel proud of yourself and your body, make it feel stronger and taller.   keep your shoulders straight and your head up even if you are 7 feet tall . Do not try to hide your height by slouching. Let the world know that you are proud of yourself and your body. that's where your soul lives , it is the home of your soul , be proud of your body and keep it in good shape by doing the right exercises daily. Make it a habit to show everyone including your mother and the whole world that you are proud of yourself and your posture, and that will make you feel good inside and out. Stand in front of a mirror , put your shoulders back, your spine straight as a pine , wing at yourself and say'' I AM PROUD OF ME AND MY POSTURE, I AM THE BEST, I can have a perfect posture with the right exercises. Put a big smile on that beautiful posture of yours and you will look like a million bucks even if you are broke. A good posture , a big smile on your face and the right attitude and you are on your way for success in anything you decide to do, both in your personal and professional life.

Lets get down to the right exercises to help you get the good posture you always wanted.

Exercise one

STANDING ON YOUR TOES.

1) STANDING ON YOUR TOES AS OFTEN AS YOU CAN.
Standing on your toes is a very good exercise for

good posture and ballerinas exercise daily to get strong feet and all the muscles of their legs for good posture. You have to start slowly   to avoid any injuries to your toes , muscles and ligaments. Use a chair or the wall to help you stand straight. Place both hands on the chair, pull your tummy in , bring your shoulders back and raise your body on your toes. You should feel tall and straight . Hold that position to the count of three and lower your feet to the ground.

Repeat it for ten times. Rest for a few minutes and do it again for ten times. Take it easy and do not overdo it. As your feet and legs muscles are getting stronger you keep increase the repetitions until you reach at least 100 repetitions.

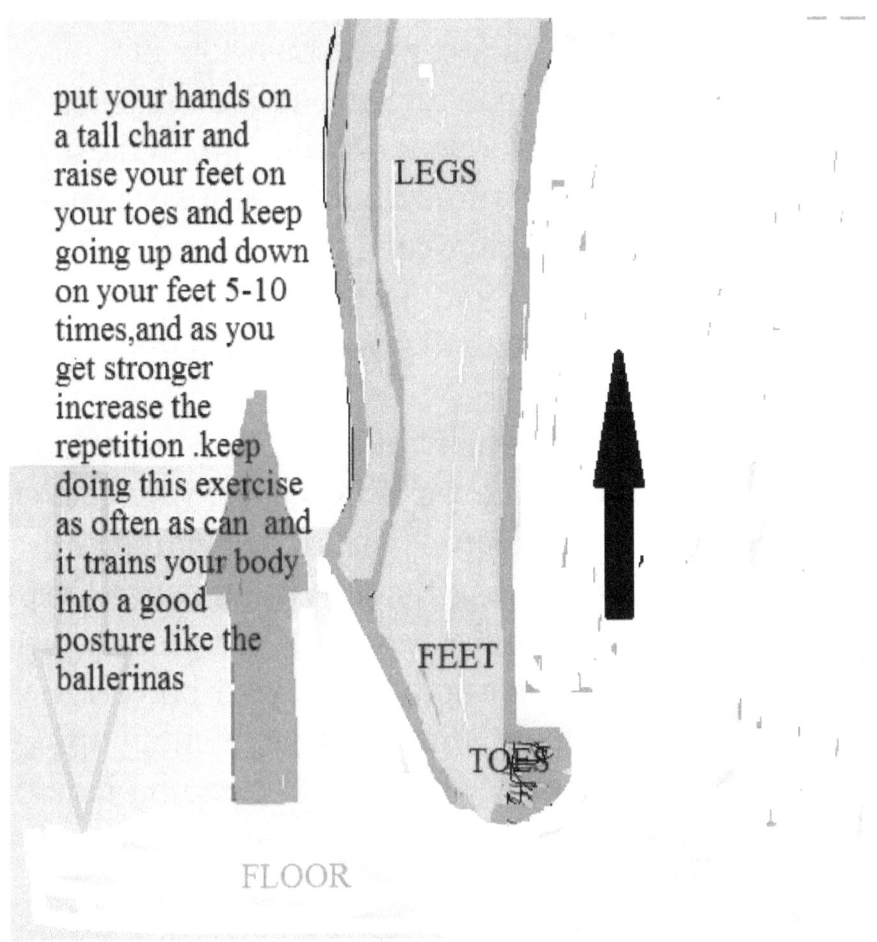

As time goes by and you get stronger you will not need the support of a chair or the wall and you will be able to do these exercises anywhere at any time. I encourage you to do them anywhere whenever you get a chance, at home, at the bus stop, at work at school . The idea is to get strong feet muscles while you do these exercises. While you do these exercises, your body is forced into a good posture and by doing it over and over again you get into the habit of keeping your body in good alignment and with time will be natural to you to have a good posture.

With This exercise , when you stand on your toes , your body is forced into a smaller base, your feet toes, and in order to keep your body standing and avoid falling down due to the gravity, it has to keep the gravity line within the new smaller base. By changing into a smaller body base your body has to re-arrange the gravity line by straightening up your body and the only way to stay standing it has to force the gravity line within the new smaller base and a straight body frame.

Anyway this is one of the best exercises for good posture and it is the cornerstone exercise of the ballerinas graceful good posture .

EXERCISE TWO

2)KNEE TO CHEST EXERCISES WHILE LYING DOWN.

You might be wondering, what does the knees to chest exercises have to do with a good posture? Well, In order to have a good posture you have to

have a strong, flexible and healthy spine. The
spine is the key for a good posture and knee to
chest exercises is one of the best exercises to keep
the spine strong, flexible and healthy. You can do
this exercise every morning and night in your own
bed, or on a small mat on your room floor.
Lie down face up,
bend your knees and bring them to your chest
about 8-12 inches apart,
Grab your knees the right knee with the right hand
And your left knee with your left hand
 and press your knees on your chest
And raise your head towards your knees
Hold this position to the count of three
Let your head down to the mat
Take a deep breath
And then raise your head towards your knees again
and hold it to the count of three.
Repeat this exercise for five times and keep
increasing the number of repetitions as you get
stronger.
THIS EXERCISE IS A SPINAL STRETCHING
EXERCISES AND STRETCHES ALL THE
VERTEBRAE OF YOUR SPINE!

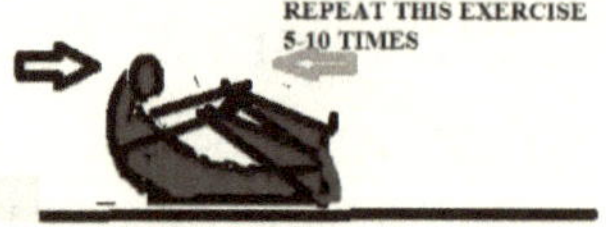

WITH YOUR KNEES BENT DRAW BOTH KNEES TO YOUR CHEST,
GRAB YOUR KNEES WITH BOTH HANDS DRAWING THE KNEES AS NEAR
TO THE CHEST AS POSSIBLE.
AND THEN RAISE YOUR HEAD TOWARDS YOUR KNEES

WITHOUT STRAINING YOURSELF

HOLD IT FOR THE COUNT OF TWO

THEN LOWER YOUR HEAD GENTLY TO THE MATTRESS
AND YOUR FEET TO THE MATTRESS

While you are lying down with your knees bent
Do the next   knees to chest rocking exercises.

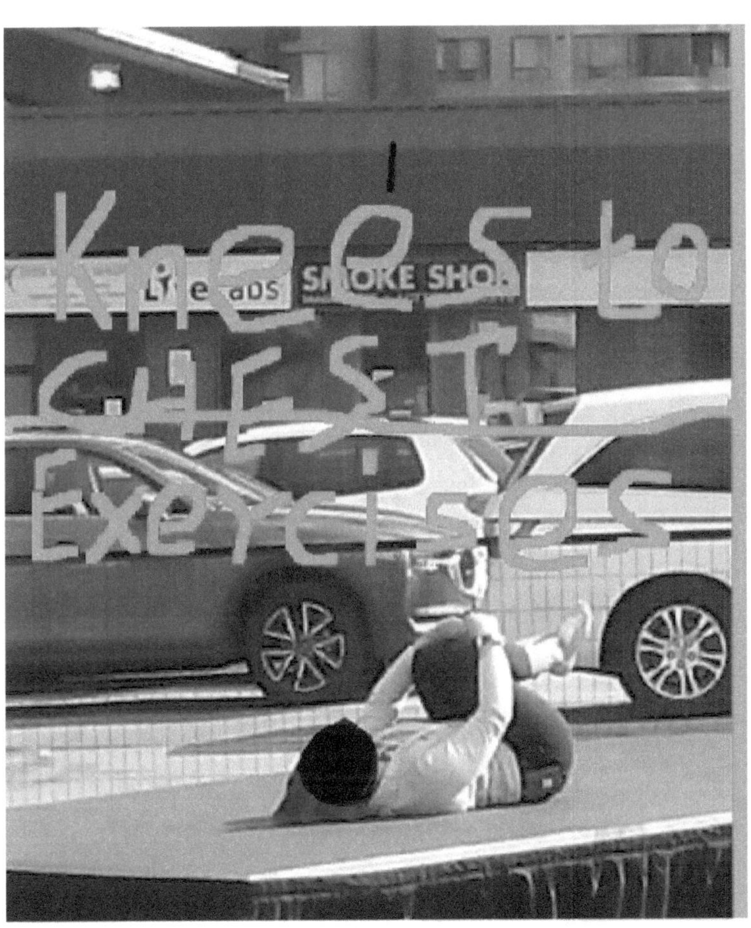
Knees to
chest
Exercises

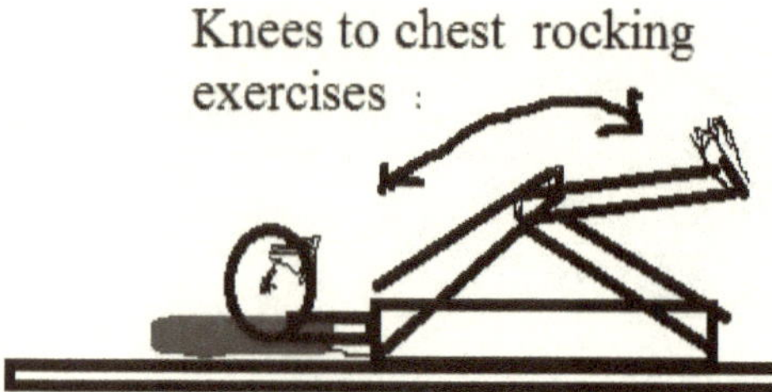

grab your right knee with your right
hand and your left knee with your left
hand and bring your knees to your
chest and with a rocking motion rock
your pelvis back and forth

These exercises are the best exercises for your
spine but you should never overdo it or strain
yourself, take it easy and go slow in the beginning
until you get stronger and more flexible.
These exercises can help flatten your stomach and
strengthen your abdominal muscles as well.

Remember to do these exercises on
an empty stomach and never after a
meal when your stomach if full.

N.B. DO NOT DO THESE EXERCISES IF YOU

HAVE ANY PATHOLOGY IN YOUR SPINE OR
IF YOU HAD SPINAL SURGERY AND RODS
IN YOUR SPINE.
 Remember to Stop doing any activity that causes
pain or makes pain worse. Pain is a warning of
your body   and you listen to your body.

EXERCISE THREE

3)INTERLOCK YOUR FINGERS AND PLACE
THEM UNDER YOUR HEAD.
While lying down face up, interlock your fingers
and place them under your head.
Take a deep breath expanding your chest as much
as possible and then exhale slowly. Repeat it for
5 times.
Then bring your elbows towards your face
And then back to the mattress pressing on the
mattress
Repeat this exercise 5 times and as you get

stronger increase them to 20-50 times.
This exercise is very good for strengthening your
shoulders and upper body muscles and ligaments.
Always start with a deep breath and exhale
slowly.

LYING FACE UP WITH FEET EXTENDED

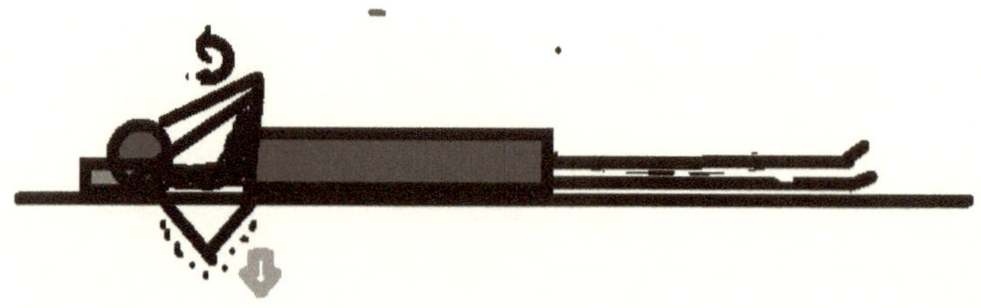

INTERLOCK YOUR FINGERS AND PLACE YOUR HANDS UNDER YOUR HEAD AND YOUR
ELBOWS TOUCHING THE MATTRESS.
THEN
BRING YOUR ELBOWS TOWARDS YOUR FACE AND THEN BACK
PRESSING ON THE MATTRESS.

EXERCISE FOUR

SPRING CHEST EXPANDERS.

4) Buy and use the spring chest expander which
is a simple piece of equipment consisting of two
handles connected by 2-5 springs that provide

resistance when you try to expand them.
Chest expanders are versatile, allowing you to perform a wide range of **exercises** in the privacy of your own home.
The spring expanders are cheap to buy and easy to use in the privacy of your home. You can buy them at the local sport shop or on line.
The name says it all, chest expanders are used to expand and strengthen your chest muscles, shoulder and arm muscles. Strong and expanded chest muscles are a good indication for a good posture. When you buy these spring chest expanders come with instructions how to use them which is a good thing. With chest expanders you can use them to exercise all body muscles. You can use some free videos on you tube how to use them properly and get the maximum benefit from using this piece of equipment.
Here I am going to describe the upper body chest exercises.
When you start out do not over do it and do not use all the springs that come with the chest expanders, start with one or two springs and as you get stronger you add more springs.

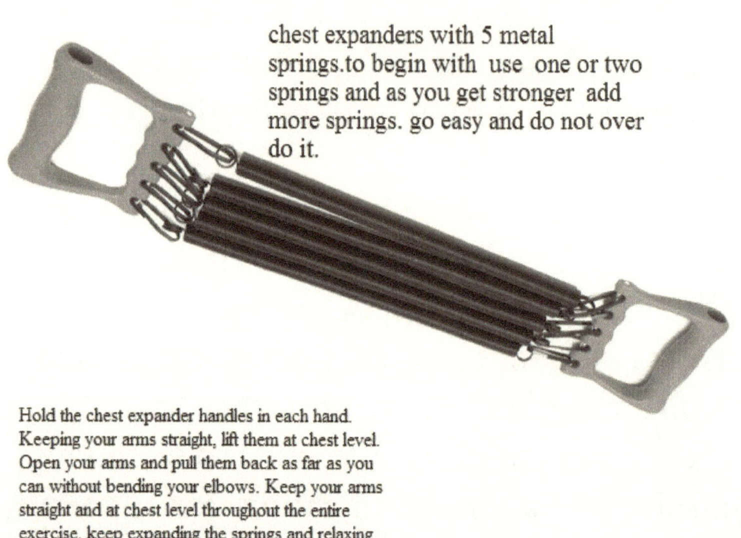

Hold the chest expander handles in each hand.
Keeping your arms straight, lift them at chest level.
Open your arms and pull them back as far as you
can without bending your elbows. Keep your arms
straight and at chest level throughout the entire
exercise. keep expanding the springs and relaxing
them. repeat for 5-10 times. rest and start over
again. do not overdo it. take it easy.

Hold each chest expander handles with your palms facing out. .keep your arms straight in front of your chest and expand them as far as you can, hold it to the count of three and then bring your straight arms in front of your chest . Repeat the same exercise 5-10 times and then rest.

You can also raise your arms   above your head and pull them back slightly so that the chest expander is positioned behind your neck at your shoulders level and pull to expand them from there to work the shoulder muscles and other muscles of your upper middle back.

You should always be careful while exercising not to loose the grip on one of the handles which can result in an injury to yourself.

You can do a lot of exercises with the chest expanders exercising the muscles of your arms, legs, shoulders etc. I am sure the   spring chest expanders come with instructions how to use them and many types of exercises you can do.
The chest expanders springs are very good to exercise your muscles and get a good posture.

Work at your own pace and strength   and do not let the springs press on your skin for your own protection against injury.

5)monkey bar   pull up exercises

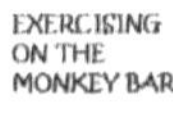

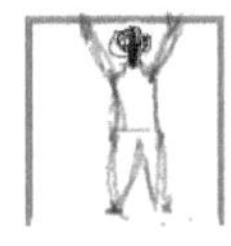

Pull Up Bar Workouts is the best upper body exercises. Not many people can do these exercises as it requires a lot of strength. Start with just holding the bar with both hands facing away from you at shoulder width apart and let your body swing back and forth. This position stretches your whole spine with your own body weight and exercises your shoulders and arms. Eventually when you get stronger you do the pull up exercises raising your chin towards the bar.

Pull up by bending your elbows until your chin clears the bar and when the chin is above the bar the upwards phase of the pull up is complete. Then ease yourself down gently and   if you feel strong enough you can pull up towards the bar again and do a few pull ups without interruption .When you finish the pull up exercises, ease yourself down gently and rest for a few minutes by taking a few deep breaths. If you feel strong enough you can do a few more pull ups .

Go easy and do not strain yourself, do one or two at the beginning and as you get stronger you increase the repetitions. Make sure the bar is strong and secure to avoid any unexpected surprises by the bar giving way and injuring you.

Pull ups are a great way to improve posture by strengthening your upper body muscles.. Pull ups work the whole upper body, the arms, shoulders, chest and stretching your spine with your own weight. This makes training on a pull up bar perfect for building upper body strength , endurance, stretching your spine and a perfect posture.

The pull ups exercises are as good as weight lifting because helps make your back straighter, open up your chest and pushing back your shoulders for a good posture, especially if have to work on a desk job and your shoulders hunch forward all day.
If you do not have access to a monkey bar you can buy some cheap 2-5 lbs weights and do some weight lifting training at home, which will help you get stronger and get a better posture. Look at all those body builders that spend a lot of time training with weights and they have a good posture. I never saw a bodybuilder with a bad posture, they all have a very good posture which is the envy of many people.

 Pull ups or in other words, lifting your body weight to a horizontal bar, achieves the same results as lifting weights . When exercising with weights it is good to concentrate on the upper body muscles especially the chest and shoulders. If you decide to do some weight lifting, It is a good idea to use a waist support while lifting weights to avoid any strain or injuries to your back.

Lifting weights and other exercises along with
eating right, especially high protein foods is the
best thing you can do for your body and posture.
Exercises and good food will give you a good
posture and good health that will be the envy of
many.

N.B. when you start a new routine of exercises
Always go easy and if you have any health
problems , consult your trusted doctor before
starting any strenuous exercises.

EXERCISE SIX

SWIMMING

6) swimming is an excellent exercise for good
posture.
 Swimming is a very good exercise to improve or
maintain your posture. With swimming you
exercise all the muscles of your body especially
your shoulders, spine and legs.
Swimming is a great workout that builds muscle
strength, endurance and cardiovascular fitness.
Make sure you know how to swim before you dive
into the water of a pool, sea or the ocean. If you do

not know how to swim, you can take lessons in your local swimming pool with an expert swimming teacher. But if you are afraid of the water , stay out of the water altogether and do other sports which are as good for your posture. Although the benefits of swimming are many, it is not worth to risk your life if you do not feel comfortable with water activities.

If you are a swimmer and you enjoy water activities make sure that the water you are about to swim in is clean and free of any toxins or bacteria that cause illnesses.

Swimming is one of the best exercises with many health benefits and you should try to swim as often as you can if you can swim, especially swimming in the open sea or ocean with salty waters..

Swimming   athletes have great postures   which is the envy of many people. It is always good to learn and benefit from the successes of others.

 If you swim during the day and the sun is too strong, it is advisable to use a hat made of cloth fabric to protect your face and head from the strong rays of the sun.

I remember one hot summer that I was swimming in the sea, I used to have a hat made of cloth fabric, like the ones the hunters use. I used to keep the hut wet to keep my head cool.

The first day I used the hat, I was the only one with a hat swimming in the sea. The next day more people wore hats while swimming and by the end of the week most of the people had hats on their heads while swimming in the sea.

It is always advisable to use a hat to protect your face and head from the strong rays of sun. Hats made of straw are ok but hats made of fabric cloth are better as you can wet the hat with cold water often, to keep your head cool.

As I said above, swimming exercises are great stretching exercises for a good posture, but if you are not a fan of swimming and the water, it is better to stay out of the water. There are lots of other great exercises that you can do on dry land to improve your posture and your health.   Swimming is the only activity for the fishes but not for all the people. And then again there are people that swim

like fishes and they love to spend endless hours of
swimming anywhere they can find water, in the
local swimming pool , the sea ,the ocean and
rivers. Good for them, maybe in their previous life,
if there is such a thing, they were fishes!

 7) WALKING TALL IMPROVES YOUR
POSTURE

AVOIDING SLOUCHING and walking tall is the
best way to improve your posture. Walking is the
basic movement we use everyday but many
people walk in a slouching position which is very
bad for the posture. Avoiding slouching when
walking will be the first step to improve your
posture. Try to walk with a good posture. Keep
your head up, your eyes forward , your shoulders
back and your palms facing your hips. Walk with a
rolling motion through your foot from heel to toe.
keep your spine straight at all times while walking.
A straight spine is the key for a good posture. You
should wear comfortable shoes to protect your feet
and make your walk easier. You should also wear
comfortable clothing and avoid tight clothing that
can make your walking difficult.
Walking with a good posture has many health
benefits. You can breath easier and protects your
musculoskeletal system from any injury or wear
and tear on your joints.

Make it a habit to walk with a good posture. Walk tall and be proud of yourself and your achievements. Never slouch while walking. With a little effort and exercises before you know it your posture will start to improve.   Keep improving day by day and you will accomplish your goal to have a good posture.

There is a Chinese proverb that goes like this " a thousand miles walk, start with the first step."   the same is true for getting a good posture. The road to a good posture starts with your first effort to walk tall and avoid slouching.

Always keep your spine straight with a good posture whether you walk, stand, sitting or running. That's the only way to improve your posture. A straight spine equals a good posture every time.

DANCING.

Besides walking ,dancing is an excellent exercise to improve your posture. You do not have to be a ballerina , a ballroom instructor or an experienced dancer, but You can have lots of fun dancing while strengthening your bones and muscles, and improving your posture and balance. Just keep your spine straight with your shoulders back and move to the music beat with your chosen partner. Dancing is just walking to the music beat and with practice you will enjoy dancing both for exercise and pleasure. Dancing on the dancing floor with someone you like is better than sitting alone on the bar drinking alcohol with the risk of getting drunk.

Dancing is a good exercise for your body and mind . Dancing will help you improve your posture while having fun.

GOOD POSTURE AND NUTRITION

A good posture requires good nutrition too. it is

absolutely necessary that you provide the essential nutrients to your body in order to have a good posture and function properly. If you do not provide good nutrition to your body, your posture and your health will pay the price. Bad nutrition and bad posture is the major cause of many health conditions, both mental and physical diseases. Nutritional deficiencies have an effect on all parts of the body. There are a lot of people that spend a lot of money for their food by they end up overfed and undernourished due to the poor choice of what they consume. When it comes to nutrition it is not how much people eat , not the quantity but the nutritional quality of the food consumed that is important.

In my book : EAT THE RIGHT FOODS FOR OPTIMUM HEALTH : by S.ELIA

Available at amazon.com , I wrote that it is very important to eat the right foods for optimum health.

So when you decide to improve your posture, I urge you to eat nutritional foods for your   body's need. When you provide your body with the necessary nutrients you will feel better, perform better and you will have a better posture. Eating right foods does wonders for your body. It is important to have a balanced diet every day so that your body function at its best. Your diet should include proteins, like meat, fish, eggs, milk, carbohydrates, fruits and vegetables so that your body gets all the nutrients necessary for good health. When you exercise, protein is the key, but you also need the vitamins and minerals found in fruits, nuts and vegetables for the body's nutritional needs. You do not have to spend a lot of money to eat well, but you have to make the right choice of foods you buy and consume. Nutritional   foods are reasonable priced and anybody can eat good food on any budget.

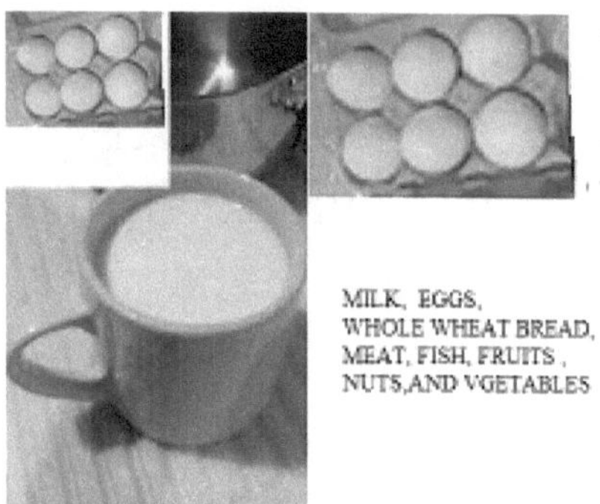

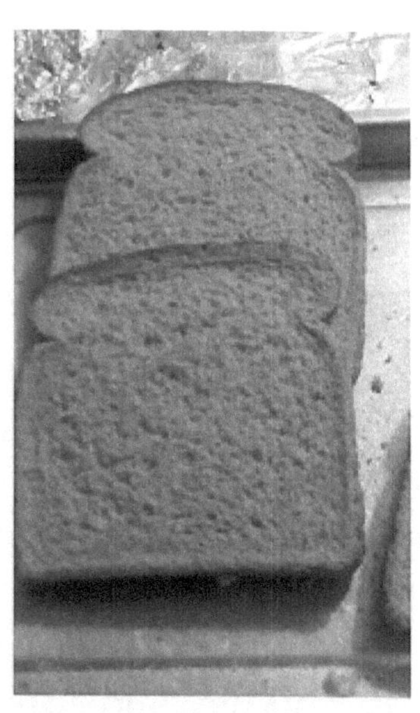

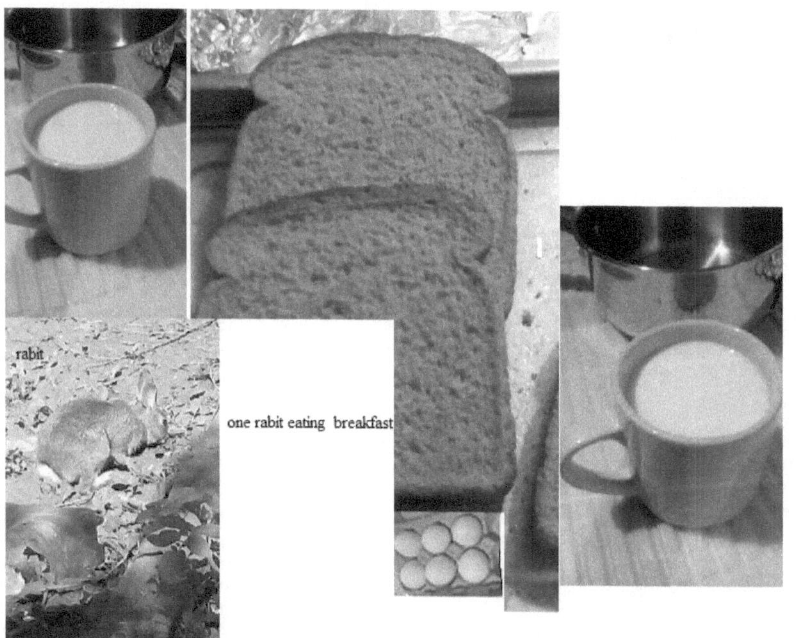

People with good posture, professional athletes, swimmers, and bodybuilders make sure to eat

nutritional foods to provide their bodies with all
the necessary nutrients for optimum health.
You do not have to overeat to supply your body
with all the nutrients needed by your body, as
overeating creates   other health problems like
obesity, shortness of breath, spinal problems , joint
problems and bad posture.
Moderation in all things including food and
exercises and your will be on your way for   better
posture.

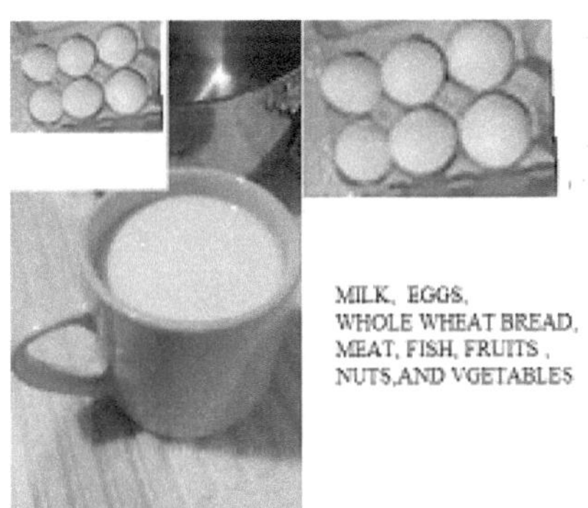

MILK, EGGS,
WHOLE WHEAT BREAD,
MEAT, FISH, FRUITS ,
NUTS,AND VGETABLES

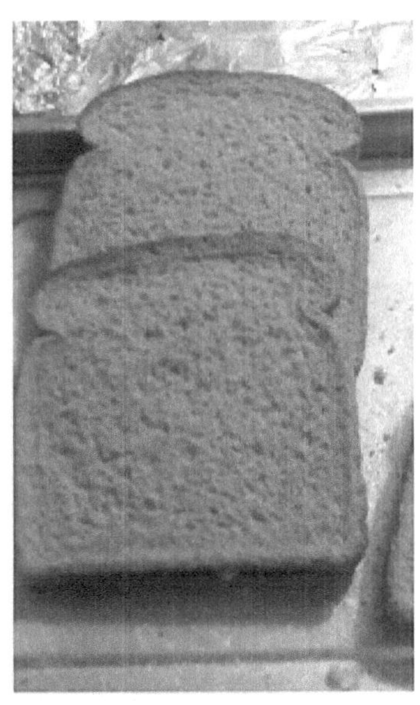

Nutritious foods for good health

Proteins is the magic key for optimum health and the most important food for repairing and maintaining your body in good shape. Eat the right foods and you will be rewarded with good health and even a long healthy life blessed with happiness and the joy of healthy living.

Eating the right foods is no more expensive that eating junk food, or wasting money on drinking alcohol, smoking, legal or illegal drugs . On the contrary nutritional foods like milk, eggs, whole wheat bread, fish   and chicken meat are reasonably priced and accessible to any budget, rich or frugal.

While we are talking about good nutrition for good health, it is important to emphasize that you should avoid substances that ruin your health, like smoking, drinking alcohol and drugs.

Avoiding these substances will help you save a lot of money too, while protecting your health from   diseases caused by these substances , like alcoholism, cancer and premature deaths from overdoses etc . The amount of money you save from avoiding the above disease causing substances, you can buy all the nutritional foods your body needs to live like a king and have more money left in your savings. It all comes down to how you use your money   and how you prioritize your budget with the money you have.

CONCLUSION

Anyone can have a good posture if they are
willing to exercise and make an effort   to
eliminate the causes of bad posture which is
slouching.
Unfortunately there is no magic pill to make
your posture perfect. If you want to have a good
posture you have to exercise daily.
   The exercises I described in this book are the best
for attaining and maintaining a good posture. All
the people that have good postures , the
professional athletes, the body builders,   the
military and the ballerinas are doing some of
these exercises daily and that's how they attained
their good postures. So if you want to have a good
posture you have to follow the examples of the
people that they already have a good posture by
doing these exercises daily. You do not have to do
all the exercises every day but if you want to be
successful   improving your posture, you have to
eliminate the slouching while you walk, standing,
sitting, running or anything else you do.

Slouching is the number one enemy of good posture and you have to give up slouching before you have a chance to improve your posture. Period.
Once the slouching is eliminated and you keep a good posture while walking, sitting or standing and you do the standing on your toes exercise ,you are halfway through to improve your posture. This is the first step to achieve your goal, a good posture.
If you can do all the exercises that's great, you can achieve your goal of a good posture sooner than later. But if you cannot do all the above exercise you have the option to choose a few of them which are the best exercises to help you achieve your goal, a good posture.
My suggestion is:
Number one : eliminate the slouching altogether in anything you do and walk with a good posture. If you cannot avoid slouching you might as well forget about a good posture.
Number two: do the standing on your toes exercises that forces your body to alignment and a good posture. Do it as often as possible, anywhere, anytime.
Number three: Do All the spinal exercises while lying down. The knees to chest for the low back exercises and your hands behind your head for

shoulder and upper back exercises.

Number four: Use the spring chest expanders which are very good to exercise your chest and upper body and any other muscle group you decide. You should try and do the chest expanders exercises daily, maybe even twice a day in the beginning. This piece of equipment will help you achieve a good posture in a short period of time when you use it properly every day.

Number five: the pull ups to a horizontal bar, and weight lifting exercises are very good for the chest and upper body muscle strength. if you have access to a horizontal bar you can do them, but this can be optional, so is the weightlifting, provided that you use the chest expanders.

Number six: swimming and dancing are excellent exercises that can help you attain a good posture, but can be optional too .

Still I recommend that you swim and dance anytime your have the time. These activities are good for your body and mind.

You decide which ones you want to do , but elimination of slouching and walking with a good posture is a must , if you really want to have a good posture.

The secret to a good posture is simple, eliminate the bad postural habits and adopt new good postural habits with exercises.

There is no short way to good posture . You have

to eliminate slouching and do the right exercises
.NOBODY ELSE CAN DO THAT FOR YOU!!
GOOD LUCK TO ALL! And may the Greek
gods bless you and your efforts with the exercises
you will be doing, to give you a great posture like
the ones the ancient Greek gods had.

Book description
  The exercises I described in this book are the best
for attaining and maintaining a good posture. All
the people that have good postures , the
professional athletes, the body builders,   the
military and the ballerinas are doing these
exercises daily and that's how they attained their
good postures. So if want to have a good posture,
you have to follow the example of the people that
they already have a good posture by doing these
exercises daily.

There is no other way to get a good posture without exercising.

Unfortunately they have not invented a magic pill yet, to take it and give you a good posture.

 You and only you can do these exercises to improve your posture.! It is your body , it is your posture and nobody else can do these exercises to improve your posture. You do not need to go to the gym or expensive equipment to give you a good posture. The only thing you need is the right exercises and exercise your body daily in the privacy of your own home.

Many people are wishing to have a good posture but they fail to do anything about it. Unfortunately, wishful thinking will never give you a good posture. If you are serious about improving your posture, you have to start doing the right exercises today, NOW, not tomorrow, not next week, not when you have the time. But right NOW! If you have the desire, will and determination to exercise daily you will achieve you desired goal. A perfect posture!

Otherwise you will be left only with your dreams and your wishful thing for a good posture.

From the inside cover.
After reading this book and attaining a good posture, give this book to someone else who needs it. Maybe a youngster you know, a friend or relative, so that he or she benefits from the exercises in this book and get a good posture too. Knowledge should be shared for the benefit all!
A candle looses nothing by lighting another candle but the room has more light from two candles instead of one.

www.ingramcontent.com/pod-product-compliance
Lightning Source LLC
Chambersburg PA
CBHW051128250726
48655CB00007B/2951